KIDNEY DISEASE

A manual guidebook
on the treatment of
kidney disease

Dr Rowan Theo

Table of Contents

CHAPTER ONE

Kidney Health and Kidney Disease Basics

What is kidney sickness?

The kidneys are a couple of fist-sized organs placed at the lowest of the rib cage. There is one kidney on every aspect of the spine.

Kidneys are important to having a wholesome frame. They are especially chargeable for filtering waste merchandise, extra water, and different impurities out of the blood. These pollutants are saved in the bladder after which eliminated in the course of urination. The kidneys additionally alter pH, salt, and potassium stages in the frame. They produce hormones that alter blood stress and manage the manufacturing of purple blood cells. The kidneys even prompt a shape of nutrition D that facilitates the frame take in calcium.

It happens whilst your kidneys emerge as broken and can't carry out their characteristic. Damage can be because of diabetes, excessive blood stress, and diverse different continual (long-time period) conditions. Kidney sickness can result in different fitness troubles, such as vulnerable bones, nerve harm, and malnutrition.

If the sickness receives worse over time, your kidneys might also additionally forestall operating completely. This method that dialysis could be required to carry out the characteristic of the kidneys. Dialysis is a remedy that filters and purifies the blood the use of a system. It can't therapy kidney sickness, however it could extend your life.

What are the kinds and reasons of kidney sickness?

Chronic kidney sickness

The maximum common shape of kidney sickness is continual kidney sickness. Chronic kidney sickness is a long-time period situation that doesn't enhance over time. It's generally because of excessive blood stress.

High blood stress is risky for the kidneys due to the fact it could boom the stress at the glomeruli. Glomeruli are the tiny blood vessels in the kidneys in which blood is cleaned. Over time, the improved stress damages those vessels and kidney characteristic starts to decline.

Kidney characteristic will ultimately go to pot to the factor in which the kidneys can not carry out their task properly. In this case, someone might want to move on dialysis. Dialysis filters greater fluid and waste out of the blood. Dialysis can assist deal with kidney sickness however it couldn't therapy it. A kidney transplant can be any other remedy choice relying for your circumstances.

Diabetes is likewise a prime reason of continual kidney sickness. Diabetes is a collection of illnesses that reasons excessive blood sugar. The improved stage of sugar in the blood damages the blood vessels in the kidneys over time. This method the kidneys can't easy the blood properly. Kidney failure can arise whilst your frame will become overloaded with pollutants.

Kidney stones

Kidney stones are any other common kidney problem. They arise whilst minerals and different materials in the blood crystallize in the kidneys, forming stable masses (stones). Kidney stones generally pop out of the frame in the course of urination. Passing kidney stones may be extraordinarily painful, however they not often reason sizeable troubles.

Glomerulonephritis

Glomerulonephritis is an irritation of the glomeruli. Glomeruli are extraordinarily small systems in the kidneys that clear out the blood. Glomerulonephritis may be because of infections, pills, or congenital abnormalities (problems that arise in the course of or quickly after birth). It regularly receives higher on its own.

Polycystic kidney sickness

Polycystic kidney sickness is a genetic sickness that reasons severa cysts (small sacs of fluid) to develop in the kidneys. These cysts can intervene with kidney characteristic and reason kidney failure. (It's essential to word that man or woman kidney cysts are pretty common and nearly continually harmless. Polycystic kidney sickness is a separate, extra critical situation.)

CHAPTER TWO

Urinary tract infections

Urinary tract infections (UTIs) are bacterial infections of any a part of the urinary system. Infections in the bladder and urethra are the maximum common. They are effortlessly treatable and infrequently result in extra fitness troubles. However, if left untreated, those infections can unfold to the kidneys and reason kidney failure.

What are the signs and symptoms of kidney sickness?

Kidney sickness is a situation that could effortlessly pass not noted till the signs and symptoms emerge as severe. The following signs and symptoms are early caution symptoms and symptoms which you is probably growing kidney sickness:

• fatigue

• trouble concentrating

• problem sleeping

• negative appetite

• muscle cramping

• swollen feet/ankles

• puffiness across the eyes in the morning

• dry, scaly skin

• common urination, specifically past due at night time

Severe signs and symptoms that would suggest your kidney sickness is progressing into kidney failure encompass:

• nausea

• vomiting

• lack of appetite

• adjustments in urine output

• fluid retention

• anemia (a lower in purple blood cells)

• reduced intercourse drive

- surprising upward push in potassium stages (hyperkalemia)

- irritation of the pericardium (fluid-crammed sac that covers the coronary heart)

What are the threat elements for growing kidney sickness?

People with diabetes have a better threat of growing kidney sickness. You will also be much more likely to get kidney sickness in case you:

• have excessive blood stress

• produce other own circle of relatives contributors with continual kidney sickness

• are elderly

• are of African, Hispanic, Asian, or American Indian descent

Learn extra: Type 2 diabetes and kidney sickness »

How is kidney sickness diagnosed?

Your medical doctor will first decide whether or not you belong in any of the excessive-threat groups. They will then run a few checks to peer in case your kidneys are functioning properly. These checks might also additionally encompass:

Glomerular filtration rate (GFR)

This take a look at will degree how nicely your kidneys are operating and decide the degree of kidney sickness.

Ultrasound or computed tomography (CT) Scan

Ultrasounds and CT scans produce clean photos of your kidneys and urinary tract. The photos permit your medical doctor to peer in case your kidneys are too small or large. They also can display any tumors or structural troubles that can be present.

CHAPTER THREE

Kidney biopsy

During a kidney biopsy, your medical doctor will put off a small piece of tissue out of your kidney even as you're sedated. The tissue pattern can assist your medical doctor decide the form of kidney sickness you've got and what kind of harm has occurred.

Urine take a look at

Your medical doctor might also additionally request a urine pattern to check for albumin. Albumin is a protein that may be exceeded into your urine whilst your kidneys are broken.

Blood creatinine take a look at

Creatinine is a waste product. It's launched into the blood whilst creatine (a molecule saved in muscle) is damaged down. The stages of creatinine to your blood will boom in case your kidneys aren't operating properly.

How is kidney sickness handled?

Treatment for kidney sickness generally specializes in controlling the underlying reason of the sickness. This method your medical doctor will assist you higher manipulate your blood stress, blood sugar, and levels of cholesterol. They might also additionally use one or extra of the subsequent strategies to deal with kidney sickness.

Drugs and medication

Your medical doctor will both prescribe angiotensin-changing enzyme (ACE) inhibitors, consisting of lisinopril and ramipril, or angiotensin receptor blockers (ARBs), consisting of irbesartan and olmesartan. These are blood stress medicines that could gradual the development of kidney sickness. Your medical doctor might also additionally prescribe those medicines to hold kidney characteristic, even in case you don't have excessive blood stress.

You will also be handled with cholesterol pills (consisting of simvastatin). These medicines can lessen blood levels of cholesterol and assist hold kidney fitness.

Depending for your signs and symptoms, your medical doctor may prescribe pills to alleviate swelling and deal with anemia (lower in the wide variety of purple blood cells).

Dietary and way of life adjustments

Making adjustments in your weight loss plan is simply as essential as taking medication. Adopting a wholesome way of life can assist save you most of the underlying reasons of kidney sickness. Your medical doctor might also additionally advocate which you:

• manage diabetes via insulin injections

• reduce returned on ingredients excessive in cholesterol

• reduce returned on salt

• begin a coronary heart-wholesome weight loss plan that consists of clean end result, veggies, complete grains, and low-fats dairy merchandise

• restrict alcohol consumption

• cease smoking

• boom bodily activity

• lose weight

Dialysis and kidney sickness

Dialysis is an synthetic approach of filtering the blood. It's used whilst a person's kidneys have failed or are near failing. Many

human beings with past due-
degree kidney sickness should
pass on dialysis completely or till a
donor kidney is discovered.

There are forms of dialysis: hemodialysis and peritoneal dialysis.

CHAPTER FOUR

Hemodialysis

In hemodialysis, the blood is pumped via a unique system that filters out waste merchandise and fluid. Hemodialysis is executed at your property or in a clinic or dialysis center. Most human beings have 3 classes in line with week, with every consultation lasting 3 to 5 hours. However, hemodialysis also can be executed in shorter, extra common classes.

Several weeks earlier than beginning hemodialysis, maximum human beings can have surgical treatment to create an arteriovenous (AV) fistula. An AV fistula is created through connecting an artery and a vein simply underneath the skin, normally in the forearm. The large blood vessel permits an improved quantity of blood to float constantly via the frame in the course of hemodialysis remedy. This method extra blood may be filtered and purified. An arteriovenous graft (a looped, plastic tube) can be implanted and used for the equal cause if an artery and vein can't be joined together.

The maximum common aspect consequences of hemodialysis are low blood stress, muscle cramping, and itching.

Peritoneal dialysis

In peritoneal dialysis, the peritoneum (membrane that traces the belly wall) stands in for the kidneys. A tube is implanted and used to fill the stomach with a fluid known as dialysate. Waste merchandise in the blood float from the peritoneum into the dialysate. The dialysate is then tired from the stomach.

There are   sorts of peritoneal dialysis: non-stop   ambulatory peritonealdialysis, in which the stomach is crammed and tired numerous instances in the course of the day, and non-stop cycler-assisted peritoneal dialysis, which makes use of a system to cycle the fluid inside and outside of the stomach at night time even as the individual sleeps.

The maximum common aspect consequences   of   peritoneal dialysis are infections in the belly hollow space or in the region in which the tube turned into implanted.   Other   aspect consequences might also additionally encompass weight benefit and hernias. A hernia is whilst the gut pushes via a weak point or tear in the decrease belly wall.

What is the long-time period outlook for a person with kidney sickness?

Kidney sickness usually does now no longer leave as soon as it's diagnosed. The quality manner to hold kidney fitness is to undertake a wholesome way of life and observe your medical doctor's advice. Kidney sickness can worsen over time. It might also additionally even result in kidney failure. Kidney failure may be life-threatening if left untreated.

Kidney failure happens whilst your kidneys are slightly operating or now no longer operating at all. This is controlled through dialysis. Dialysis entails the usage of a system to clear out waste out of your blood. In a few cases, your medical doctor might also additionally advocate a kidney transplant.

How can kidney sickness be prevented?

Some threat elements for kidney sickness — consisting of age, race, or own circle of relatives history — are not possible to manage. However, there are measures you could take to assist save you kidney sickness:

• drink masses of water

• manage blood sugar when you have diabetes

• manage blood stress

- lessen salt intake

- cease smoking

Be cautious with over the counter pills

You need to continually observe the dosage commands for over the counter medicines. Taking an excessive amount of aspirin (Bayer) or ibuprofen (Advil, Motrin) can reason kidney harm. Call your medical doctor if the regular doses of those medicines aren't controlling your ache effectively.

Get examined

Ask your medical doctor approximately getting a blood take a look at for kidney troubles. Kidney troubles normally don't reason signs and symptoms till they're extra advanced. A fundamental metabolic panel (BMP) is a preferred blood take a look at that may be executed as a part of a recurring clinical exam. It assessments your blood for creatinine or urea. These are chemical substances that leak into the blood whilst the kidneys aren't operating properly. A BMP can come across kidney troubles early, whilst they're less difficult to deal with. You need to be examined yearly when you have diabetes, coronary heart sickness, or excessive blood stress.

Limit sure ingredients

Different chemical substances to your meals can make contributions to sure forms of kidney stones. These encompass:

• immoderate sodium

• animal protein, consisting of pork and chicken

• citric acid, discovered in citrus end result consisting of oranges, lemons, and grapefruits

• oxalate, a chemical discovered in beets, spinach, candy potatoes, and chocolate

Ask approximately calcium

Talk in your medical doctor earlier than taking a calcium supplement. Some calcium dietary supplements were connected to an improved threat of kidney stones.

THE END